FERTILITY DIET

Guide for maintaining good health and preventing ongoing infections

Teresa J. Huebner

Table of Contents

INTRODUCTION

The study of what food means to the body and the connection between food and well-being is known as sustenance. It is essential for maintaining good health and preventing ongoing infections because it is a complicated and growing field. The fundamental principles of nutrition that should be understood in order to make well-informed dietary choices are referred to as "nutrition basics."

Preamble to sustenance basics incorporates securing an

understanding of the central enhancements that the human body needs to work suitably. Carbs, proteins, fats, nutrients, and minerals are instances of these supplements. Vitamins and minerals are involved in a variety of bodily functions, fats are essential for insulation and energy storage, and proteins are required for the construction and repair of tissues. Energy is provided by carbohydrates.

In addition to comprehending the essential nutrients, it is essential to understand the concept of energy balance. The equilibrium that exists between the calories obtained from food and those expended from physical activity and other bodily functions is referred to as "energy balance." When you consume more calories than you burn, you gain weight, while when you lose weight, you consume fewer calories than you burn. Understanding energy balance is fundamental for keeping a strong weight and preventing progressing contaminations like heftiness and type 2 diabetes.

By and large, understanding the job that food plays in keeping up with great wellbeing requires an establishment in sustenance. It involves comprehending the concept of energy balance and the essential nutrients required for bodily functions in order to maintain a healthy weight. People can make well-informed dietary choices that will improve their health and prevent chronic diseases if they are aware of these essential standards. Food is an essential part of our daily lives and plays a significant role in maintaining our overall health. It's more important than ever for women trying to conceive to eat well. The meaning of genuine food for productivity could never be more critical, as it can generally

impact a woman's ability to get
pregnant and pass a strong
pregnancy on to term.

CHAPTER1

Meaning of fertility

Eating a well-balanced diet that includes a variety of foods from all food groups is essential for fertility. A diet deficient in nutrients can result in erratic menstrual cycles, making it challenging for a woman to conceive. Moreover, an eating routine that is high in dealt with food assortments, sugar, and bothersome fats can provoke disturbance in the body, which can unfavorably impact extravagance. A diet high in fruits, vegetables, whole grains, lean proteins, and healthy fats is essential for fertility support.

Getting the right nutrients is also important for the health of the developing fetus. During pregnancy, a woman's body requires additional enhancements to help the turn of events and improvement of the youngster. During pregnancy, a diet deficient in essential supplements can increase the risk of birth defects and complications. To ensure the health of both the mother and the unborn child, women must eat well before and during pregnancy.

In conclusion, adequate nutrition is necessary for both fertility and the health of the developing fetus. Ladies attempting to imagine need to eat an even eating routine that incorporates various food varieties from all nutrition types. A well-balanced diet can help you control your menstrual cycles, lower inflammation, and have a better chance of getting pregnant. Our diets have a significant impact on our health and play an important role in our daily lives. During pregnancy, it may also aid in the baby's growth and development, lowering the risk of birth defects and other issues. It is especially important for pregnant women. Fundamental supplements play a crucial role in richness because they are the building blocks of healthy food. To increase their chances of becoming pregnant, women should eat a variety of essential nutrients.

CHAPTER2

Essential nutrient for fertility

Folic corrosive is one of the fundamental supplements that is significant for ripeness. The growth of the baby's neural tube requires folate, a B vitamin. To reduce the risk of birth defects, pregnant women should take no less than 400 micrograms of folic acid on a regular basis. Food sources like braced oats, verdant green vegetables, citrus products, and beans contain folic corrosive.

Another essential nutrient for fertility is iron. Iron is essential for the production of red platelets and aids in the delivery of oxygen to the infant. Consuming 27 milligrams of iron per day is recommended for pregnant women. Iron can be found in foods like beans, sustained grains, red meat, poultry, fish, and so on.

Lastly, essential nutrients include omega-3 fatty acids that improve fertility. Omega-3 unsaturated fats are a type of fat found in fish like salmon, sardines, and tuna. They can work on the nature of the egg and sperm and aid chemical guideline. Pregnant women should aim to eat at least two servings of fish per week to get the recommended amount of omega-3 fatty acids.

In conclusion, essential nutrients are necessary for fertility, so women trying to conceive should try to include them in their diet. Folic acid, iron, and omega-3 fatty acids are three essential nutrients that can assist you in becoming pregnant. If women consume these nutrients, they can have a healthier pregnancy and improve their overall health. It is essential to consult a medical services provider to determine the appropriate dosage of essential nutrients for each individual.

Sustenance altogether affects richness, as well as on broad wellbeing and prosperity. If you want to think about it, you need to pay attention to what you eat and make sure your eating habits are good for you. The right foods can help you get pregnant more often while the wrong foods can hurt fertility. Thus, keeping up with great regenerative wellbeing requires eating the fitting food sources.

New soil products are one of the most important food sources to incorporate into a richness-friendly diet. Numerous essential vitamins and minerals can assist you in becoming pregnant from these foods. For instance, leafy green vegetables like spinach and kale are high in folate, an essential vitamin for a healthy fetal development. In a similar vein, organic fruits and vegetables like mangoes, oranges, and berries are rich sources of L-ascorbic acid, which has been shown to protect eggs from harm and improve sperm quality.

Whole grains are another important group of nutrients for fruitfulness. Whole grains like oats, brown rice, and quinoa have fiber that can help control hormones and make you more sensitive to insulin. They are also a good source of important nutrients like iron and vitamin B, which can help improve reproductive health. Therefore, replacing refined grains like white bread and pasta with whole-grain alternatives is essential to support fertility.

In the end, incorporating sources of lean protein into your ripeness-appropriate diet is crucial. Protein helps build and repair tissues in the body, so it is necessary for healthy eggs and sperm to develop. Therefore, it is essential to incorporate vegetables, lean meats, fish, and eggs into your daily diet. These food sources likewise contain a ton of supplements like zinc, which can assist with directing periods and work on the nature of sperm.

Overall, a ripeness-friendly diet should include a variety of food sources high in nutrients that support mental health. Fresh vegetables, whole grains, and sources of lean protein are some of the most important foods to include in your diet if you want to conceive. By making these dietary changes, you can support a healthy pregnancy and increase your chances of getting pregnant.

With regards to fruitfulness, the meaning of nourishment couldn't possibly be more significant. Food is an important part of life. Avoiding some food sources that can hinder fruitfulness can make fruit even more ripe. To start, avoid processed foods for better fertility. This kind of food has a lot of sugar, salt, and bad fats, which can make your hormones different and make you look tired. Additionally, processed food sources contain additives, additional substances, and synthetics that can harm the regenerative framework.

CHAPTER3

Understanding how food affects our conceptual health

Dairy items high in fat ought to be stayed away from as the subsequent food. Ovulation may be disrupted by these products' high levels of saturated fats. In addition, they might make the body itch, which could make it hard to conceive. Low-fat dairy items like skim milk, low-fat yogurt, and cheddar are suggested instead of high-fat dairy items.

The third food to avoid for improved fertility is soy-based products. Phytoestrogens in soy can carry on like estrogen in the body. Consuming too much soy can cause hormonal imbalances and disrupt ovulation. It is recommended to confine soy-based things and pick various wellsprings of protein, similar to incline meat, fish, and vegetables.

In conclusion, adequate nutrition is crucial to increasing fertility. Avoiding processed foods, fat-laden dairy products, and soy-based products can improve fertility. Instead, a healthy diet rich in whole grains, lean protein, and fruits and vegetables is recommended. Changing one's diet can help one become more fertile and have a better chance of conceiving.

Understanding how food affects our conceptual health is important because food varieties and ripeness are interconnected. Our ripeness is additionally affected by the food we eat. A healthy and well-balanced diet is essential for increasing fertility. Eating a diet rich in nutrients, vitamins, and minerals can help regulate hormones and increase the chance of conception.

Certain foods have been found to increase fertility. Berries, salad greens, nuts, and seeds, which are all high in cell reinforcements, can assist with protecting the regenerative framework from free extreme harm. Omega-3 unsaturated fats, which are tracked down in salmon and other greasy fish, can likewise uphold ovulation and lessen aggravation, the two of which can further develop fruitfulness. Whole grains like brown rice, quinoa, and oats are high in fiber, which helps keep hormones and blood sugar in check, which in turn helps fertility.

Contrarily, certain foods should be avoided due to their potential to affect fertility. Trans fats, high-sugar handled food varieties, and irritation, insulin opposition, and hormonal irregular characteristics all adversely affect richness. Smoking, excessive alcohol consumption, and caffeine consumption can all have a negative impact on fertility. It is essential to limit or avoid these habits in order to increase fertility.

In conclusion, a nutritious and well-balanced diet is necessary for increasing fertility. Ripeness can be improved by remembering food varieties high for omega-3 unsaturated fats, cell reinforcements, and fiber. In a similar vein, avoiding foods that can affect fertility, such as processed foods, sugar, trans fats, caffeine, and alcohol, can also help improve reproductive health. Talking to a doctor and a registered dietitian can help you create a fertility-friendly diet plan.

Supplements that support fruitfulness can be found in abundance in salad greens. These greens contain vitamins and minerals that can improve your reproductive health. The focus on show that mixed greens like spinach, kale, and collard greens have more folate, which is important for a healthy fetal development. Folate also aids in the prevention of birth defects and miscarriage.

CHAPTER 4

Benefits of some food to help reduce problem in the body

In addition to containing foliate, leafy greens also contain iron, which is necessary for maintaining healthy blood levels. Hemoglobin, the protein in red platelets that conveys oxygen to your tissues, is made to a great extent with iron. Iron deficiency can lead to frailty, which can cause fatigue, shortcoming, and other health problems. Regular consumption of salad greens can help prevent frailty and ensure that your body receives the oxygen it needs to function properly.

One more clinical benefit of salad greens is their ability to reduce exacerbation in the body. Inflammation can make fertility problems and other issues with the reproductive system worse. Cell reinforcements in salad greens assist with lessening irritation and keep up with great wellbeing. By eating more leafy greens, inflammation can be reduced and reproductive health can be improved. Increasing your intake of leafy greens can generally improve fertility and reproductive health.

It has been demonstrated that certain foods increase the likelihood of conception, which in turn improves fertility. Nuts are one of these food sources. Nuts aren't just a tasty snack; they also have a lot of nutrients that can help people get pregnant.

Nuts contain a lot of healthy fats, protein, and fiber, all of which are important for good reproductive health. They additionally contain various nutrients and minerals, including zinc, magnesium, and vitamin E, which are all fundamental for ripeness. Magnesium, then again, can assist with managing chemicals and further develop glucose levels, and vitamin E is a cell reinforcement that can assist with safeguarding the regenerative framework from hurt. Then again, the creation of solid sperm and eggs relies upon zinc.

Research has moreover shown the way that eating nuts can help with chipping away at the idea of sperm and eggs. Compared to men who did not consume nuts, those who did had better sperm motility, morphology, and count. A study that was published in the journal Nutrients revealed this. It was also discovered that women who consumed nuts on a regular basis had better egg quality and a greater likelihood of origination.

By and large, nuts are an unprecedented development to any readiness helping diet. They are easy to integrate into feasts and tidbits, and as well as upgrading richness, they can have various other positive wellbeing impacts. However, you need to be careful about how much you eat because nuts have a lot of calories and can make you gain weight if you eat too many of them. Therefore, if you're looking for a sound tidbit, you might want to go after a small handful of nuts to help your ripeness.

Fertility and overall health require a well-balanced diet and whole grains. Whole grains are rich in fiber, vitamins, and minerals that help maintain a healthy weight, reduce inflammation, and regulate hormones, all of which are essential for increasing fertility. Whole grains are an extraordinary wellspring of many-sided carbs, which give the truly important energy expected to consider and convey a sound pregnancy.

Whole grains like oats, brown rice, quinoa, and barley, which are high in essential nutrients like foliate, iron, and zinc, are known to improve fertility in both men and women. Folate is essential for healthy fetal development and can prevent neural tube defects in babies. Zinc is important for sperm motility and creation, and iron guides in oxygen transport all through the body, including the conceptive framework. It has been demonstrated that consuming whole grains on a regular basis significantly boosts fertility and the likelihood of a healthy pregnancy.

It's important to remember that not all grains are created equal. The high glycemic index of refined grains like white bread, pasta, and rice has the potential to cause insulin resistance, which can lead to weight gain and hormonal imbalances. On the other hand, whole grains have a lower glycemic index, which helps control blood sugar, reduce inflammation, and make insulin more sensitive. Include whole grains in your daily diet to boost fertility and overall health.

CHAPTER5

The role of diet in fertility
And food to stay away from

Diet plays an important role in promoting fruitfulness. A healthy diet that includes a variety of supplements can help people of all ages grow their fruitfulness further. Consuming foods that help you conceive is a safe and natural way to improve your reproductive health.

Foliate is one of the most important nutrients for good health. This B vitamin prevents birth defects and enhances sperm quality. Folate can be found in fortified grains, citrus fruits, beans, and leafy greens. Omega-3 unsaturated fats are also essential for ripening because they improve egg quality and increase blood flow to the embryonic organs. Incorporate flaxseeds, chia seeds, and pecans in your eating routine, as well as slick fish like salmon, sardines, and mackerel.

An additional nutrient that is necessary for fertility is zinc. Zinc helps to regulate hormone levels and increases sperm motility and count. Zinc can be found in oysters, beef, pork, poultry, beans, and nuts. Because they protect the conceptive cells from oxidative damage, cancer prevention agents like L-ascorbic acid and vitamin E are also important for richness. To boost your consumption of cell reinforcement, include berries, organic citrus products, nuts, and seeds in your diet.

In general, a diet high in whole foods and well-balanced is necessary for fertility. Combining readiness assisting food assortments with loving plate of mixed greens, smooth fish, beans, nuts, and seeds can chip away at your potential outcomes envisioning ordinarily. Keep in mind that drinking alcohol, eating processed foods, and drinking sugary drinks can harm your reproductive health. With the help of a nutritionist or dietitian, a custom meal plan that boosts fertility can be created.

Diet is one of numerous things that can influence ripeness, which is a confounded issue. While some foods can make it harder to get pregnant, others can help. It is essential to be aware of the food sources you should avoid, assuming you are trying to imagine. We'll look at some of the foods you shouldn't eat if you want more developed richness in this article.

Handled meats are one of the food sources you should avoid assuming you are attempting to imagine. Additives and added substances found in handled meats like wieners, frankfurters, and store meats can adversely affect fruitfulness. Furthermore, these meats much of the time contain a ton of soaked fat, which can cause irritation in the body. If inflammation prevents ovulation and implantation, it can make it harder to conceive.

Sweet beverages are another food you ought to stay away from for better richness. Sweet drinks like pop, caffeinated drinks, and improved teas can make people gain weight, which can make fruit less likely to ripen. Women who are overweight or obese are more likely to experience difficulty getting pregnant and to have irregular menstrual cycles. Drinking sugary beverages can also make you insulin resistant, making it harder to conceive and less fertile.

Finally, you should avoid food sources that are high in trans fats accepting you are endeavoring to consider. Margarine, baked goods, fried foods, and processed foods typically contain trans fats. It is common knowledge that these fats raise inflammation levels in the body, which may impede implantation and ovulation. In addition, trans fats have the potential to make you insulin-resistant and cause you to gain weight, both of which can make it more difficult to conceive.

All in all, being aware of what you eat is fundamental assuming that you are attempting to imagine. For better fertility, avoid processed meats, sugary drinks, and foods high in trans fats. You can increase your chances of considering and having a healthy pregnancy by choosing healthy foods and maintaining a healthy weight.

Richness necessitates a well-being-based diet. Women who are trying to imagine need to pay close attention to what they eat and stay away from particular types of food. Inadequate nutrition can disrupt ovulation, fertilization, and even implantation. Specialists in the field of ripeness say that pregnant ladies ought to eat different good food sources and avoid those that can hurt fruitfulness.

Handled food sources are one of the main things to stay away from when trying to think about them. Processed foods are loaded with unhealthy fats, salt, and sugar. Irritation brought about by these food varieties can influence fruitfulness. Conceptive organs can be harmed and, surprisingly, the nature of eggs and sperm can be impacted by aggravation. Therefore, processed foods should be avoided at all costs.

Another food that shouldn't be eaten when trying to conceive is caffeine. Caffeine can make it harder for the body to absorb certain supplements, like iron, which is essential for fruitfulness. Infertility is more common in women who drink a lot of caffeine than in women who don't. Therefore, the recommended daily limit for caffeine consumption is one or two cups of coffee.

Last but not least, avoiding alcohol is essential when trying to conceive. The hormonal balance, ovulation, and even the nature of sperm can all be disrupted by alcohol. According to studies, women who consume alcohol frequently take longer to reflect than those who do not. Therefore, it is recommended to completely avoid alcohol when trying to conceive. In conclusion, it is essential to eat a well-balanced diet and avoid foods that can hinder fertility when trying to conceive. Avoiding certain foods can have negative effects on fertility. One of these is handled food sources, which can make it hard for someone to think clearly. Types of handled food are those that have undergone some form of modification from their original structure, typically through the addition of artificial flavors, additives, or other synthetics. These sorts of food sources are generally speaking high in calories, sugar, and lamentable fats, all of which can add to unproductiveness.

One of the primary negative effects that processed foods have on fertility is how they affect body composition and weight. Weight gain, which can have an effect on hormonal balance and ovulation, can be caused by the high calorie content of many processed foods. Additionally, the body may become irritated as a result of these foods, which may have a greater impact on fertility. A diet high in processed foods can also lead to insulin resistance, which can cause irregular periods and other fertility issues.

The general well-being of processed food sources is another negative effect on wealth. Handled food varieties frequently lack vitamins and minerals, increasing the risk of chronic diseases like diabetes, heart disease, and obesity. All of these conditions have the potential to make it harder to conceive and reduce fertility. By focusing on a diet high in whole, nutrient-dense foods and avoiding processed foods, people can improve their overall health and increase their chances of conception.

When everything is taken into account, avoiding handled food sources is a crucial step for anyone who wants to improve their productivity. Weight, hormonal equilibrium, and in general wellbeing can be in every way harmed by these food sources, making it more testing to consider. By focusing on a diet high in whole, nutrient-dense foods, people can support their overall health and well-being and increase their chances of conception.

Foods to Avoid: How Alcohol Use Affects Fertility Alcohol use can have a big impact on a person's health and is common in many social settings. However, alcohol consumption can also have an impact on fertility, particularly in women. Numerous studies show that drinking alcohol frequently can change hormone levels and disrupt ovulation, affecting fertility. Drinking alcohol while pregnant can also make it more likely that the baby will have birth defects or a miscarriage. Therefore, women trying to conceive should completely avoid consuming alcohol.

Besides, it is imperative to observe that the impact of alcohol usage on productivity isn't limited to women. Men who regularly consume alcohol may experience fertility issues as a result of low sperm count and quality. This is because of the way that liquor can modify the development of testosterone and different chemicals, diminishing the amount and nature of sperm. Erectile dysfunction, which can have a negative effect on fertility, can also be caused by alcohol use. Thus, keeping away from liquor utilization is exhorted for all kinds of people attempting to imagine.

In conclusion, drinking alcohol can have a significant impact on both men's and women's fertility. Regular alcohol consumption can cause hormonal imbalances, ovulation issues, a lower sperm count, and erectile dysfunction. Drinking alcohol while pregnant can also cause stillbirths and birth defects. As a result, people trying to conceive should cut back on alcohol or completely avoid it. Prioritizing one's health and well-being is essential when trying to start a family

Caffeine, a stimulant, can be found in chocolate, tea, coffee, and some soft drinks. It can altogether affect our wellbeing and is one of the substances that is consumed the most universally. A growing body of research suggests that excessive caffeine consumption can have a negative impact on fruitfulness.

Because it can prevent the production of chemicals that are necessary for ovulation to take place, caffeine consumption may have an impact on wealth. Additionally, caffeine has the potential to restrict blood flow to the uterus, making it more difficult for an undeveloped organism to embed. Caffeine utilization can influence sperm motility and lower sperm quality by and large in men.

It is recommended that you limit your caffeine intake to 200 milligrams per day if you are trying to conceive. This is equivalent to two cups of tea or one cup of coffee. Caffeine consumption should also be avoided at all costs during the early stages of pregnancy because it can increase the likelihood of an unanticipated labor.

Overall, while drinking caffeine is generally safe for most people, taking a lot of it can hurt wealth, especially in people trying to think. If you're trying to think, it's important to watch your caffeine intake and drink only moderate amounts. You can increase your chances of conception and have a healthier pregnancy by doing this.

CHAPTER6

Recipes and meal planning

Recipes and meal preparation are important aspects of a healthy lifestyle, especially for people trying to conceive. Extravagance is a confounding cycle that can be impacted by diet and different elements. People trying to conceive may benefit from knowing how to plan meals that boost fertility.

When planning meals for fertility, put nutrient-dense foods first that help maintain hormonal balance and overall health. This recollects food sources high for malignant growth anticipation specialists, sound fats, and micronutrients like zinc and vitamin D. It's furthermore basic to keep away from dealt with and sweet food assortments since they can disturb synthetic harmony and make the body more leaned to aggravation.

Fertility-supporting dishes can be delicious and simple to prepare. Examples of feasts that are excellent for ripeness include quinoa and dark bean salad, lentil soup with kale, and broiled salmon with vegetables. These recipes consolidate upgrade thick decorations that help efficiency, like omega-3 unsaturated fats, fiber, and iron. In addition, these dishes can be altered to meet specific dietary requirements and preferences.

In conclusion, recipes and meal planning are useful resources for couples trying to conceive. Keeping up with hormonal equilibrium and generally speaking wellbeing can be kept up with by zeroing in on thick food sources and staying away from handled and sweet food varieties. Recipes that are good for fertility can be tasty and easy to make, making meal planning fun and helpful during the process of getting pregnant.

It may become a priority for people who want to increase their wealth and health as well as their health. As a result, it's critical to think about the ways that the foods we eat can affect our health in a variety of ways, including when they are ripe. Knowing how certain foods and dietary patterns may affect fertility outcomes is important because nutrition plays a significant role in fertility.

When it comes to food and wealth, there are a few important considerations to make. A significant idea is that body weight affects fertility. In order to maintain a healthy weight, it is essential to eat a well-balanced and nutritious diet because being overweight or underweight can affect fertility. Vitamin D, iron, and folic acid, among other nutrients, have been shown to improve fertility. Consuming these supplements can assist you with getting pregnant and keep up with great regenerative wellbeing all in all.

It is significant for revolve around eating a moved and changed diet that integrates a ton of food sources developed from the beginning, proteins, and sound fats to additionally foster readiness through food. In addition, advancing richness and solid propagation depend on whole grains like quinoa and brown rice. In addition, it's important to limit the amount of handled and sweet food you eat because they can affect how richness turns out. Individuals can assist in maximizing their chances of conceiving and having a healthy pregnancy by focusing on a diet high in the nutrients that support fertility and overall health.

Recipes and planning a feast are essential for maintaining a healthy lifestyle. A healthy eating plan that incorporates regular foods, vegetables, lean proteins, whole grains, and healthy fats is essential. People have begun to focus on meal planning and preparation that is beneficial to fertility as the rate of infertility has increased. A healthy diet can support fruitfulness and make it more likely that seeds will be produced.

Organizing the dinner and laying the groundwork for readiness includes coordinating clear food sources that are essential to conceptual prosperity. It includes foods rich in antioxidants, vitamins, minerals, and other nutrients that control hormones, reduce inflammation, and improve the health of eggs and sperm. Whole grains, nuts, seeds, fatty fish, leafy greens, and berries are all foods that help with fertility. Trans fats, sugary drinks, processed foods, and other foods with trans fats should all be avoided at all costs because they are all bad for fertility.

Various food varieties that furnish the body with the vital supplements ought to be all remembered for an eating routine that is helpful to fruitfulness. In order to maintain stable blood sugar levels, it is suggested that you consume three to four meals per day with snacks in between. Protein, complex sugars, healthy fats, and fiber should all be present in a balanced meal. For a productive dinner, attempt quinoa bowls with avocado and seared vegetables, salmon with sweet potato and asparagus, and lentil soup with entire grain bread. Organizing a feast and getting ready for it can be difficult, but by coordinating the right food options, it can help cut down on most of the wealth and improve the chances of success.

Recipes and planning a feast are necessary for smart dieting. They enable individuals to extend their overall prosperity and preserve their stamina and energy. Regarding their richness, a few recipes can help you get pregnant more frequently. These recipes can help women improve their fertility, maintain a healthy weight, and rebalance their hormones.

Meals that support the reproductive system and aid in the formation of healthy eggs are included in recipes for optimal fertility. Antioxidants, vitamins, minerals, and healthy fats are frequently present in these recipes. Sugar and handled food varieties, the two of which can possibly cause aggravation and hormonal irregular characteristics, are missing from their weight control plans. Roasted vegetables, whole-grain pasta with tomato sauce, and lean meats like fish or chicken are examples. These meals have a lot of nutrients in them and may help women keep a healthy weight, which is important for getting pregnant.

A smoothie bowl made with avocado, salad greens, and berries is another recipe for optimal readiness. This recipe has a lot of nutrients, minerals, cancer-fighting agents, and healthy fats. Vitamin C, which improves the quality of eggs, is abundant in berries. Avocados contain sound fats that can assist with keeping up with chemical equilibrium. Leafy greens contain a lot of nutrients that can reduce inflammation and improve the reproductive system's overall health.

In conclusion, meal preparation and recipe creation are necessary for a healthy lifestyle. For women trying to conceive, recipes that promote optimal fertility may mean the difference between success and failure. Fertility, hormone balance, and reproductive system support are the goals of these recipes. Ladies can adopt a proactive strategy to their richness interaction and increment their possibilities winning by joining recipes like smoothie bowls made with berries, blended greens, and avocado or entire grain pasta with pureed tomatoes, stewed vegetables, and lean protein.

Dinner arranging and readiness can be a troublesome undertaking for some individuals, yet with the right direction, it can turn into a wonderful and calm insight. The most crucial thing to remember is preparation. Plan your meals for the week from the get-go around the start of the week. As well as aiding you in going with better food choices, this will help you with making opportunity and money. While arranging your banquets, remember your timetable and plan appropriately. For instance, if you have a busy day ahead of you, prepare for a simple, quick blowout that doesn't take up any time.

One more basic hint for convincing dinner coordinating and organizing is to make a staple once-finished and stick to it. You will actually want to keep up with your course and try not to settle on hurried decisions. When you make your basic food list, be sure to include all of the ingredients you'll need to make your meals. Additionally, this will assist you in avoiding multiple weekly grocery store visits. Additionally, if the circumstances permit, you might want to consider purchasing in bulk because doing so could ultimately save you money.

Last but not least, planning a feast requires being efficient and well-organized. One helpful tip is to prepare your ingredients ahead of time. For example, you can marinate meat or slash vegetables ahead of time. This will save you time when you plan dinners. Also, consider adding a lazy cooker or a second pot for easy and helpful gala preparation. These gadgets can help you save time and put on wonderful galas with little effort, which is a win-win situation.

In conclusion, a few straightforward suggestions can simplify meal planning and preparation. You can eat healthier and save money by planning ahead, making a list of what to buy, and preparing meals in a timely and organized manner. Meal planning and preparation can become a stress-free and enjoyable experience with a little effort and a few useful tools.

THE END

www.ingramcontent.com/pod-product-compliance
Lightning Source LLC
Chambersburg PA
CBHW050749260726
48661CB00001B/494